Table of Contents

PREVIEW

The bones of the skeletal system serve many important functions for the body, from giving your body support to allowing you to move. They also play an important role in blood cell production and fat storage.

Bone marrow is the spongy or viscous tissue that fills the inside of your bones. There are actually two types of bone marrow:

BONE MARROW DIET RECIPES

BREAKFAST

1. Braaied Mielie Atchar

Prep Time: 20 Minutes

Cook Time: 10 Minutes

Servings: 6

Ingredients

- 4 cobs sweetcorn
- 1 small red pepper, diced
- ½ cup extra virgin olive oil
- ½ cup white wine vinegar
- 1 T pickle masala
- 1 T paprika
- 1 t ground fenugreek
- 2 bird's-eye chilies
- 2 T brown sugar
- 1 medium onion, diced
- 10 g fresh coriander, roughly chopped
- Sea salt and freshly ground black pepper, to taste

Instructions

1. Heat a grill and roast the sweetcorn until well charred, but not burnt. Slice the kernels off the cob and place in a bowl.

2. Add the remaining ingredients and combine well. Pour into sterilized jars and seal. Refrigerate once cooled. Store for two days before use to develop flavor.

2. Panettone Granola

Prep Time: 20 Minutes

Cook Time: 40 Minutes

Servings: 5

Ingredients

- 100 g panettone, cubed
- 360 g rolled oats
- 1 orange, zested
- 100 g Woolworths mixed seedless raisin selection
- 1 t salt
- 100 g raw almonds, roughly chopped
- 32 g chia seeds
- 1 t almond essence
- 1/3 cup extra virgin olive oil
- 100 g caster sugar

Instructions

1. Preheat the oven to 120°C. Line a baking sheet with baking paper and grease lightly. Place the panettone

onto the baking sheet and bake for 10 minutes, or until slightly dried and crisp. Set aside.

2. Combine the remaining ingredients in a bowl. Place on a baking sheet, turn up the oven to 180°C and bake for 30 minutes, stirring occasionally, until golden brown. It will still be soft when you remove it from the oven, but will crisp up as it cools.

3. Once cooled, mix with the panettone and store in a clean, dry, airtight container.

3. Green Salad with Goat's Cheese

Prep Time: 10 Minutes

Cook Time: 00 Minutes

Servings: 4

Ingredients

For the dressing, mix:

- 1 T sherry vinegar
- 3 T olive oil
- 5 g Italian parsley, chopped
- Sea salt and freshly ground black pepper, to taste
- 100 g bag Woolworth's baby spinach, rocket and watercress
- 2-3 stick celery, thinly sliced
- 100 g dried cranberries
- 35 g Woolworth's nut and seed sprinkle
- 2 x 100 g logs Woolworth's chevin
- 2 avocados, quartered
- Sea salt and freshly ground black pepper, to taste

Instructions

1. Place the salad leaves in a bowl. Pour over the dressing
    and toss gently.
2. Top with the celery, cranberries, nut and seed sprinkle,
    chevin and avocado. Season to taste.

4. Loaded Potatoes 2 Ways

Prep Time: 10 Minutes

Cook Time: 40 Minutes

Servings: 4

Ingredients

- 4 Kara orange sweet potatoes
- 2 Theresa spice blend

Olive oil:

- Sea salt and freshly ground pepper, to taste

Meaty option:

- 100 g chorizo coins, fried
- 100 g Woolworths South African feta & spiced Cheddar cubes with chickpeas cheese pot
- Micro leaves, to garnish

Meat-free option:

- 1 avocado
- ½ lemon, juiced
- Sea salt and freshly ground pepper, to taste

- 2 T plain yogurt
- ¼ cup water
- 100 g South Africa feta, mozzarella, hard cheese with seed and herbs cheese pot
- Watercress, to garnish

Instructions

1. Slice potatoes in half lengthways drizzle with olive oil and coat with the spice blend.
2. Microwave on high for 8-10 Minutes until par cooked.
3. Wrap each half in tin foil and place over hot coals, turning every few minutes to avoid burning. They will cook for 20 -25 minutes over the coals.
4. Sprinkle with feta cheese pots and top with fried chorizo coins for the meaty version. For the meat-free version, blend together avocado, lemon juice, yoghurt and water until smooth. Season. Top braaied sweet potatoes with avocado mixture and top with feta, mozzarella, hard cheese with seed and herbs cheese pot.

5. Baby Marrow Fritter Bowl

Prep Time: 20 Minutes

Cook Time: 15 Minutes

Servings: 6

Ingredients

- 2 x 260 g pun nets Woolworths green pesto and bulgur wheat salad
- 175 g pun net Woolworth's green summer crunch salad
- ¼–½ cup olive or canola oil, for frying
- ½ cup plain double-cream yoghurt
- 1 T Woolworths harissa paste
- 125 g Woolworths yellow exotic tomatoes, sliced
- 4 red spring onions, sliced
- For the baby marrow fritters:
- 500 g baby marrows, grated
- 1 free-range egg
- 3 T flour
- 1 lemon, zested
- 1 t thyme, chopped
- Sea salt and freshly ground black pepper, to taste

Instructions

1. Mix the two readymade salads.

2. To make the baby marrow fritters, combine all the
    ingredients in a bowl. Cover and chill for 30 minutes.

3. Heat the oil in a large pan over a medium heat.
    Carefully drop tablespoonful of batter into the hot oil,
    taking care not to overcrowd the pan. The mixture will
    be slightly loose, but it will stick together as it hits the
    oil. Fry until golden, turn and fry the other side. Drain
    on kitchen paper and repeat with the remaining batter.

4. Mix the yoghurt and harissa, place in a small bowl and
    drizzle with olive oil.

5. Top the salad with the fritters, tomatoes and spring
    onions. Drizzle with the dressing.

6. Sweetcorn Potato Salad

Prep Time: 20 Minutes

Cook Time: 30 Minutes

Servings: 4

Ingredients

- 700 g pack Woolworths microwave baby potatoes with garlic butter
- 2 t Woolworths Cape Malay curry spice
- Sea salt and freshly ground black pepper, to taste
- 2 T olive oil
- 2 cobs sweetcorn, kernels removed
- 1 head radicchio (or use Woolworths' Italian salad leaf mix)
- 10 g coriander
- 1 red onion, thinly sliced

For the coconut-and-coriander dressing:

- ½ can coconut milk
- 1 lime, juiced
- 15 g coriander
- 1 green chili, chopped

- Salt, to taste

Instructions

1. Preheat the oven to 220°C. Cook the potatoes according to package instructions. Place on a baking tray with the butter from the pack and gently squash using the back of a fork. Sprinkle with the Cape Malay spice, salt and drizzle with olive oil. Roast for 20 minutes or until crispy and golden.
2. To make the dressing, place all the ingredients into a blender and blend until smooth. Spread the dressing onto a large platter just before assembling the salad.
3. Scatter the potatoes and remaining ingredients onto the dressing. Serve warm.

7. Chuckles rusks

Prep Time: 2hrs 5 Minutes

Cook Time: 40 Minutes

Servings: 24

Ingredients

- 750 ml buttermilk (no buttermilk?
- 215 g butter, melted
- 20 g dry yeast (2 sachets)
- 95 g sugar (1/2 cup)
- 1 t salt
- 1 t bicarbonate of soda
    - kg organic stone ground cake flour (or a mix of 700 g cake flour and 700 g white bread flour)
- 2 x 250g bags Chuckles

Instructions

1. Combine the buttermilk, melted butter and yeast in a large mixing bowl (or the bowl of a mixer) and stir until the yeast starts to dissolve and bubble slightly.

2. Add the sugar, salt and bicarbonate of soda and mix well.

3. Add two thirds of the flour to the liquid mixture and stir until combined. If you're using an electric mixer, use the dough hook.

4. Add more flour while mixing and kneading until the mixture comes together to form a workable dough. If the dough feels right, don't add more flour.

5. Fold 250g Chuckles into the dough. Place the dough in a lightly oiled bowl, loosely place a piece of plastic wrap directly on the dough and cover it with a damp cloth. Leave, in a warm area, to rise to double the original volume. It will take about 1 hour.

6. When it's done rising, shape the dough into even golf ball-sized portions. Roll them neatly and pack them tightly together in a single layer in a greased baking tray or bread loaf tin.

7. Stud the buns with the remaining Chuckles, pushing them in gently.

8. Cover with a damp cloth and leave to rise until doubled in size. This will take about 45 minutes. Preheat oven to 180°C.

9. When the final proofing is done, bake the dough for 30-40 minutes until golden brown and cooked through.

Leave to cool down just enough to work with. You can eat them at this point as fluffy buns, but if you want to turn them into rusks, break the cooked dough into pieces along the lines of the original balls, lay out flat on baking sheets and leave in an oven heated to 100°C overnight or until completely dry, at least 8 hours.

8. Mosbolletjie Rusks

Prep Time: 00 Minutes

Cook Time: 25 Minutes

Servings: 3

Ingredients

For the Mosbolletjie rusks:

- 250 g butter, at room temperature
- 320 g white sugar
- 1 x 385 g can condensed milk
- 5 eggs
- 5 kg cake flour
- 15 ml salt
- 30 g instant yeast
- 50 g aniseeds
- 1 liter lukewarm water

For the sugar syrup:

- 80 g white sugar
- 50 ml water

Instructions

3. To make the Mosbolletjie rusks

1. Cream the butter and sugar together in a large bowl. Add the condensed milk and mix.

2. Add the eggs, one at a time, beating well after each addition.

3. In a separate very large bowl, sift the cake flour and salt together. Mix in the yeast and aniseeds.

4. Add the lukewarm water to the egg and butter mixture and stir gently.

5. Add the wet ingredients to the dry ingredients and knead the dough well for about 5 minutes.

6. Place the dough in a very large, oiled bowl. Cover well with Clingfilm and leave in a warm place (not too warm as it will kill the yeast) to prove until doubled in volume.

7. Knock down the dough and shape it into balls (golf ball size, about 80 g each).

8. Place the balls in three large, well-greased loaf tins, packed tightly.

9. Leave to rise once again – it must at least double in volume.

10. Preheat the oven to 180 °C.

11. Place the tins in the oven and bake for 10 minutes. Lower the oven temperature to 160 °C and bake for 20 minutes until golden brown and cooked.

9. ClemenGold rusks

Prep Time: 20 Minutes

Cook Time: 40 Minutes

Servings: 24

Ingredients

- 2 ClemenGolds
- 4 cups water
- 2 cups buttermilk
- 200 g butter, melted
- 20 g instant dry yeast (2 sachets)
- 1 T vanilla extract
- 100 g brown sugar
- 1 t salt
- 1 t bicarbonate of soda
- 1½ kg cake flour
- 100 g Woolworths white chocolate drops

Instructions

1. Boil the ClemenGolds in the water until softened, about 10 minutes, then purée until smooth but with a bit of texture.

2. Combine the buttermilk, ClemenGold purée, butter and yeast in a large mixing bowl (or the bowl of a stand mixer) and stir. Allow to stand until the yeast starts to dissolve and bubble slightly. Add the sugar, salt and bicarbonate of soda and mix well.

3. Add two-thirds of the flour and stir until combined. If you're using an electric mixer, use the dough hook.

4. Add more flour while mixing and kneading until the mixture comes together to form a workable dough. If the dough feels right, don't add more flour. Add the white chocolate drops and combine well.

5. Place the dough in a lightly greased bowl, loosely place a piece of plastic wrap directly on the dough and cover it with a damp cloth. Allow to prove for 1 hour, or until doubled in size.

6. Once the dough has risen, shape it into even portions. Roll into balls and pack tightly in a single layer in a greased baking tray or loaf tin, almost like tiny rolls or mosbollletjies. Cover with a damp cloth and prove once

again until doubled in size. This will take about 45 minutes.

7. Preheat the oven to 180ºC. Bake for 30–40 minutes, or until golden brown and cooked through. Allow to cool just enough to work with. Once cooled, gently separate the rusks and place on a baking tray. Reduce the oven's temperature to 90ºC. Slowly dry your rusks out in the oven overnight or for 7 hours. They will be crisp and ready for dunking the very next day! Serve with hot tea.

10. All-bran rusks

Prep Time: 20 Minutes

Cook Time: 55 Minutes

Servings: 25

Ingredients

- 500 g butter
- 370 g sugar
- 500 ml buttermilk
- 1 ml lemon juice
- 3 large free-range eggs
- 1 kg self-rising flour
- 2 t baking powder
- 1 t salt
- 240 g All-bran wheat flakes
- 100 g oats (uncooked)
- 100 g pecan nuts or almonds

Instructions

1. Preheat the oven to 200°C.

2. Melt the butter and let it cool down then beat the eggs, sugar and buttermilk into the melted butter. Sift the self-rising flour, baking powder and salt together.

3. Add the All-Bran, uncooked oats and pecan nuts. Combine the wet ingredients with the dry.

4. Pour into a large oven pan (330 x 280 mm), lined with foil or baking paper and bake for 25 minutes.

5. Reduce the heat to 180°C for another 25 minutes or more, until golden brown.

6. Cool slightly before turning out and let it cool down.

7. Slice into slices and then cut into fingers. Place the fingers on a drying rack and dry in your oven at 80°C until the rusks are dry, crunchy and brittle. Once they've cooled down, place them in an air tight container.

LUNCH

11. Rusk Queen Of Puddings

Prep Time: 30 Minutes

Cook Time: 30 Minutes

Servings: 6

Ingredients

- 1 liter milk
- 500 g Woolworth's buttermilk rusks, broken into pieces
- 1 lemon, zested
- 1 ClemenGold, zested
- 1 T butter
- 6 free-range egg yolks, separated
- 300 g Bonne Maman raspberry jam
- 180 g caster sugar

Instructions

1. Preheat the oven to 180°C. Bring the milk to the boil in a saucepan over a medium heat. Remove from the heat

and stir in the rusks, lemon and ClemenGold zest and butter. Cool for 20 minutes.

2. Lightly beat the egg yolks and add them to the cooled rusk mixture. Pour the mixture into a 22 cm pie dish. Bake for 15 minutes, or until set. Remove from the oven and allow to cool. Spread the raspberry jam all over the pudding.

3. Beat the egg whites using an electric mixer until soft peaks form. Slowly add the caster sugar, a little at a time, and beat until the meringue is stiff and glossy. Spoon the meringue over the pudding and return to the oven to cook for 10 minutes, or until the meringue is golden.

12. Bresaola

Prep Time: 15 Minutes

Cook Time: 00 Minutes

Servings: 2

Ingredients

For the brine:

- 1.5 liters red wine
- 1½ T glucose
- 2 T honey
- 2 star anise
- 2 t black peppercorns
- 2 T fine salt
- 1 T pink salt
- 2 T dark brown sugar
- 1 lemon, halved
- 1 orange, halved
- 5 juniper berries

For the beef:

- kg beef topside

Instructions

1. Mix all the brine ingredients in a large plastic container.
2. Add the meat and soak in the brine in the fridge for 10 days.
3. Remove the meat from the brine, pat dry and wrap in muslin cloth.
4. Leave to hang for six weeks in the fridge.
5. After six weeks, it's ready for slicing. Serve with bread, salads or as cold meat.

13. Braaied sirloin

Prep Time: 5 Minutes

Cook Time: 15 Minutes

Servings: 2

Ingredients

- 600 g x 1 sirloin steak
- 2 T canola oil
- 4 T butter
- Sea salt and freshly ground black pepper, to taste
- 2 T Dijon mustard

For the slaw:

- 5 radishes, thinly sliced
- 1 green apple, thinly sliced
- 2 celery sticks, thinly sliced
- 1 baby green cabbage, thinly sliced
- ½ cup coconut yoghurt
- 2 T fish sauce
- Salt, to taste

Instructions

1. Allow the steak to come to room temperature. Brush with canola oil and braai over hot coals for 5 minutes per side, then rest for 10 minutes.
2. To make the slaw, toss all the ingredients together.
3. Heat the butter in a pan on the braai until browned. Drizzle the steak with the brown butter, season and serve with the mustard and slaw.

14. Sorghum-And-Bean Chili

Prep Time: 5 Minutes

Cook Time: 60 Minutes

Servings: 2

Ingredients

- 50 g Woolworths red sorghum, soaked overnight
- 50 g dried speckled beans, soaked overnight
- 2 cups stock or water
- 4 T olive oil
- 200 g lean beef mince
- 1 small onion, roughly chopped
- 1 bird's-eye chili, chopped
- 1 clove garlic, finely chopped
- 1 T Woolworths steak rub
- 1 t ground cumin
- 1 t ground coriander
- 1 t dried oregano
- 100 g diced canned tomatoes, (freeze the rest!)
- 2 T crème fraiche, for serving
- 1 baby onion, finely chopped, for serving
- 10 g Cheddar, grated, for serving

Instructions

1. Drain the sorghum and beans, place in a saucepan and cover with the water or stock. Cook for 40 minutes, or until the beans are cooked. Drain, reserving the cooking liquid.
2. Heat the olive oil in a separate saucepan and fry the mince until cooked, about 5 minutes. Add the onion and chili.
3. Fry gently for 5 minutes, or until the onion is soft and well caramelized. Add the garlic and spices and fry for 2 minutes, or until fragrant.
4. Add the tomatoes, sorghum, beans and their cooking liquid and stir until well combined. Simmer uncovered for 10 minutes, stirring occasionally. When the sauce is reduced and thick, stir once more. Serve topped with the crème fraiche, onion and cheese.

15. Beef Cheek Hand Pies

Prep Time: 15 Minutes

Cook Time: 3hrs 2 Minutes

Servings: 4

Ingredients

- ½ cup olive oil
- 600 g beef cheeks (or short rib
- Sea salt and freshly ground black pepper, to taste
- 1 stick celery, roughly chopped
- 1 large onion, roughly chopped
- 1 large carrot, peeled and roughly chopped
- 2 cloves garlic
- 1 liter beef stock
- 4 T soya sauce
- 2 T brown sugar
- 1 sheet Woolworths frozen puff pastry, thawed
- Flour, for dusting
- 1 free-range egg, beaten
- 2 T Szechuan pepper, coarsely ground

Instructions

1. Heat half the olive oil in a large saucepan. Season the meat and brown, about 3 minutes.

2. Add the celery, onion, carrot and garlic and fry until soft.

3. Stir in the stock, reduce the heat and simmer for 2½ hours, or until the meat falls apart easily. Add a little water if necessary.

4. Remove the meat from the saucepan, reserving the liquid, and place in a bowl. Shred using two forks.

5. Heat the remaining olive oil in a separate pan. Add the meat, soya sauce, sugar and ½ cup of the cooking liquid and simmer for 10 minutes, stirring occasionally. Remove from the heat and cool completely.

6. Preheat the oven to 180°C. Flour a work surface and roll out the pastry. Using a 10 cm bowl as a guide, cut out circles using a sharp knife. Remove any excess pastry and freeze to use another time. Place a heaped spoonful of meat into the center of each pastry circle and fold in half. Crimp the edges using a fork, making sure to pinch out all the air.

7. Prick the surface of each pie once. Line a baking sheet with baking paper, place the pies on the baking sheet

and brush with the egg. Sprinkle with the Szechuan pepper and bake for bake for 12–15 minutes, or until golden brown. Serve with a dipping sauce.

16. Oxtail Osso Buco

Prep Time: 35 Minutes

Cook Time: 4hrs 60 Minutes

Servings: 8

Ingredients

- 300 g Woolworths Angus beef chuck
- 1.3 kg oxtail
- 1 T flour
- 1 T flour
- 1 t salt
- 1 t white pepper
- 4 T olive oil
- 3 t butter
- 1 onion, chopped
- 2 leeks, chopped
- 2 sticks celery, chopped
- 2 carrots, chopped
- 4 bay leaves
- 3 sprigs rosemary
- 6 sprigs thyme
- 2 T tomato paste

- 1 x 410 g can diced tomatoes
- 1 cup rosé wine
- 4 cups beef stock
- Sea salt and freshly ground black pepper, to taste
- Polenta or risotto, for serving
- For the gremolata, toss
- 2 t lemon zest
- 20 g Italian parsley, finely chopped
- 1 clove garlic, finely chopped

Instructions

1. Preheat the oven to 160°C. Toss the oxtail and chuck in the flour, salt and pepper.
2. Heat the olive oil and butter in a large cast-iron or ovenproof pan that has a lid. Brown the meat until golden, then remove from the pan.
3. Add the vegetables and herbs and sauté until soft and golden. Add the tomato paste, tomatoes, wine and stock. Return the meat to the pan and bring to the boil.
4. Cover tightly with greaseproof paper and tin foil and cover with the lid. Place in the oven and cook for 5 hours. Season to taste. 5 Sprinkle with the gremolata and serve with polenta or risotto.

17. Braaied Beef Fillet

Prep Time: 15 Minutes

Cook Time: 45 Minutes

Servings: 4

Ingredients

- 800 g Woolworths free-range beef fillet
- Sea salt and freshly ground black pepper, to taste
- Olive oil, for searing

For the braai basting, mix:

- ½ cup soya sauce cup
- 2 red chilies, seeded and chopped
- ¼ cups honey
- 3 T canola oil

Instructions

1. Season the fillet and rub in olive oil. Sear all over on a very hot braai until golden brown and a crust starts to form – resist the urge to keep turning it over.

2. Remove from the heat and pour the basting over the fillet as it rests. Just before you're ready to serve,

1. Place it back on the braai and baste the meat until sticky and catching slightly but not burning.

2. When cooked to your liking, remove from the heat and allow to rest for 10 minutes. Slice, dress with basting sauce and serving with the salad.

18. Double-Smoked Salmon Dip

Prep Time: 10 Minutes

Cook Time: 00 Minutes

Servings: 8

Ingredients

- 300 g Woolworth's hot-smoked salmon fillet with pepper and dill
- 250 g mascarpone
- 1/2 lime, juiced
- 2 T soya sauce
- 2 T milk
- 1 t sriracha
- 2 T fresh dill, chopped, plus extra to garnish
- 100 g smoked salmon, thinly sliced, for serving
- 1/2 stick celery, cut into lengths, for serving
- 1 Mediterranean cucumber, peeled, cored and cut into sticks, for serving
- Woolworth's beetroot chips, for serving

Instructions

1. Blend the salmon, mascarpone, lime juice, soya sauce, milk, sriracha and dill until smooth and creamy.
2. Make salmon roses with the smoked salmon.
3. Transfer the dip into a serving bowl and garnish with chopped dill and the salmon roses.
4. Arrange on a platter with the celery, cucumber and beetroot chips.

19. Roast Cauliflower with Chimichurri

Prep Time: 15 Minutes

Cook Time: 20 Minutes

Servings: 4

Ingredients

- 1 T coriander seeds
- 1 T cumin seeds
- 5 cardamom pods, crushed
- 4 garlic cloves, finely grated
- Salt, to taste
- Extra virgin olive oil, to coat
- 350 g cauliflower florets

For the chimichurri dressing, mix:

- 1 red onion, finely chopped
- 4 T coriander roughly chopped
- 3 T parsley roughly chopped
- 1/2 red chili, finely chopped
- 1/2 green chili, finely chopped
- 1/2 cup red wine vinegar
- 1 lime, zested and juiced

- 3 T extra virgin olive oil
- 2 T brown sugar

Instructions

1. Preheat the oven to 180°C. In a large mixing bowl, combine the coriander and cumin seeds, cardamom, garlic and salt, then add the olive oil and cauliflower. Toss to coat.
2. Place the cauliflower in a roasting dish and roast for 30 minutes, or until tender and slightly charred.
3. Transfer to a serving dish and top with the chimichurri dressing.

20. Hot-Sauce Pork

Prep Time: 15 Minutes

Cook Time: 30 Minutes

Servings: 4

Ingredients

For the marinade, mix:

- 2 T honey
- 2 T soya sauce
- 3 T Tabasco sauce
- 2 T sriracha sauce
- 1 t dried chili flakes
- 2 T sunflower or peanut oil
- 700 g pork fillet
- 2 T sunflower oil
- 1 t ginger, crushed
- 1 t garlic, crushed
- 1 red chili, chopped
- ¼ cup teriyaki sauce
- 300 g Brussels sprouts, blanched and chopped

Instructions

1. Toss the pork in the marinade and marinate overnight or for at least 30 minutes. Preheat the oven to 180°C.
2. Heat 1 T oil in a large ovenproof pan and fry the pork over a high heat, then roast for 15 minutes. Set aside.
3. Using the same pan, heat the remaining oil and add the remaining ingredients. Stir-fry for 4 minutes. Slice the pork and serve with the Brussels sprouts.

DINNER

21. Bacon-And-Egg Fried Chipotle Rice

Prep Time: 15 Minutes

Cook Time: 20 Minutes

Servings: 4

Ingredients

- 2 T olive oil
- 1 onion, finely chopped
- 250 g Woolworths diced bacon
- 1 T garlic, crushed
- 100 g Woolworths whole chipotle chilies in adobo sauce, chopped
- 500 g rice, cooked
- 4 free-range eggs
- 3 T chili oil
- Coriander, to garnish

Instructions

1. Heat the oil in a large pan. Fry the onion over a medium heat until soft, then add the bacon and cook through. Add the garlic and cook for 1 minute.
2. Add the chipotles and cook for 1 minute, then add the rice and stir until coated.
3. Heat the chili oil in a separate pan and fry the eggs. Serve the rice topped with the eggs and garnish with coriander

22. Apricot Harissa Roast Chicken

Prep Time: 15 Minutes

Cook Time: 1hr 15 Minutes

Servings: 4

Ingredients

- 1 free-range chicken
- 4 T olive oil
- 1 x 140 g Woolworths apricot harissa, jar
- Salt, to taste
- 6 shallots, halved (or 3 onions, quartered)
- 1 x 400 ml coconut cream, can
- ¾ cup chicken stock

Instructions

1. Preheat the oven to 180°C. Rub the oil and harissa all over the chicken and season with salt. Place the chicken in a baking dish. Pour in the coconut milk and stock, then cover with foil and roast for 1 hour. Remove the foil and roast for a further 15 minutes.

2. Remove from the oven and rest for 15 minutes before
serving.

23. Deep-Fried Pickles on Flatbread

Prep Time: 20 Minutes

Cook Time: 20 Minutes

Servings: 5

Ingredients

- 120 g flour
- 1 t baking powder
- 1 t Woolworths Cajun seasoning
- 1 free-range egg
- 1 cup milk
- 120 g panko breadcrumbs
- Sunflower oil, for frying
- 6 halved Woolworth's jalapeño cones in brine
- 12 Woolworths sweet-and-sour sliced gherkins
- Lemon or lime wedges, for serving

For the flatbread:

- 140 g flour
- ½ t salt
- 1 cup full-cream yoghurt

For the avocado dressing, blend:

- 1 avocado, peeled and stoned

- 15 g coriander, chopped

- 15 g chives

- 2 T Woolworths sliced jalapeños in smoke-flavored brine

- 2 garlic, cloves

- 1 cup buttermilk

- Salt, to taste

Instructions

1. Whisk the flour, baking powder, Cajun seasoning, egg, and milk. Heat the oil in a large saucepan.

2. Pat dry the pickles with kitchen paper. Dip into the batter, then lightly into the breadcrumbs. Lay on a tray for about 5 minutes so the crumbs stick, then fry in batches until light brown. Drain on kitchen paper.

3. To make the flatbread, mix all the ingredients and bring together to form a ball using your hands. Wrap in cling-wrap and chill for 30 minutes.

4. Divide the dough into 6 pieces and roll out on a floured surface. Heat a griddle pan and pan-fry on both sides for a few minutes.

5. To serve, pile the pickles onto the flatbreads and drizzle
    with the dressing. Serve with lemon or lime wedges.

24. Parmesan-And-Anchovy Meatballs

Prep Time: 20 Minutes

Cook Time: 35 Minutes

Servings: 3

Ingredients

- 500 lean beef mince
- 120 g breadcrumbs
- 2 cloves garlic, crushed
- 1 t dried parsley
- 50 g Parmesan, grated
- 1 lemon, zested
- Sea salt and freshly ground black pepper, to taste
- 6 anchovies, finely chopped
- Oil, for frying

For the gravy:

- 1 T butter
- 1 T olive oil
- 4 shallots, roughly chopped
- 1 red onion, roughly chopped
- 2 cloves garlic, crushed

- 1 T flour
- 2 cups beef stock
- 3 T Worcestershire sauce
- 1 t lemon juice
- Salt, to taste

Instructions

1. Preheat the oven to 180°C. Combine the meatball ingredients and roll into 10 balls. Pan-fry the meatballs in the oil in a heavy-based saucepan until golden brown.
2. To make the gravy, heat the butter and olive oil in a pan. Fry the shallots, red onion and garlic until soft.
3. Mix the flour and stock, add to the pan and reduce for 20 minutes. Season with Worcestershire sauce, lemon juice and salt. Pour the gravy over the meatballs and bake for 10 minutes.

25. Roast Cauliflower with Cheese Sauce

Prep Time: 15 Minutes

Cook Time: 45 Minutes

Servings: 4

Ingredients

- 2 heads cauliflower, blanched for 2 minutes
- 3 T, plus 1 t olive oil
- Sea salt and freshly ground black pepper, to taste
- 140 g Woolworth's ruby mixed leaves

For the cheese sauce:

- 2 T butter
- 1 T flour
- 1 cup milk
- Salt, to taste
- 50 g Parmesan, grated
- 20 g Cheddar, grated
- 20 g mozzarella, grated

Instructions

1. Preheat the oven to 180°C. Place the cauliflower on a baking tray, drizzle with olive oil and season. Roast for 25 minutes, or until golden brown, then grill for 5 minutes.
2. Meanwhile, make the cheese sauce. Melt the butter in a small saucepan over a medium heat, then add the flour. Cook, while whisking, until browned. Gradually whisk in the milk and cook until thick and smooth. Add the cheese and stir gently until melted, then season.
3. Remove the cauliflower from the oven. Heat 1 t olive oil in a large pan and quickly sauté and season the leaves.
4. Serve the cauliflower on the leaves topped with the cheese sauce and extra Parmesan.

26. Pistachio-And-Duck Stuffing Bacon-Wrapped Terrine

Prep Time: 20 Minutes

Cook Time: 40 Minutes

Servings: 8

Ingredients

- 1 x 250 g pack Woolworths streaky wood-smoked bacon
- 1 x 600 g pack Woolworths duck sausages
- 1 T olive oil
- 3 - 4 bulbs baby fennel, chopped
- 2 t Woolworths prepared roasted garlic
- 8 fresh sage leaves, chopped
- 1/2 Woolworths ciabatta, torn into bite-sized pieces
- 100 g dried cranberries
- 1 orange, zested and juiced (optional)
- 100 g raw shelled pistachios
- Sea salt and freshly ground black pepper, to taste
- 1 large free-range egg, beaten
- Honey, for brushing

Instructions

1. Preheat the oven to 180°C. Line a 28 x 7 x 9 cm loaf tin with baking paper, then line the paper with the bacon so the sides and base of the tin are completely covered.

2. Snip the ends off the sausages and squeeze out the sausage meat. Heat the olive oil in a pan and fry the sausage meat until browned. Add the fennel, garlic and sage and fry for 5 minutes. Fold in the ciabatta.

3. Remove the pan from the heat and mix in the cranberries, orange juice and zest and pistachios. Season to taste. Fold through the egg.

4. Press the mixture into the bacon-lined loaf tin and level. Fold over any overhanging bacon pieces. Roast for 20 minutes, or until set. Remove from the oven and allow to cool to room temperature.

5. Just before serving, carefully turn out the terrine onto a baking tray, brush with the honey and place under the grill for 1–2 minutes, or until sticky and glazed. Take care not to let it burn. Slice and serve with your favorites roast.

27. Easy Peanut Butter Garage Noodles

Prep Time: 10 Minutes

Cook Time: 15 Minutes

Servings: 4

Ingredients

For the peanut butter dressing:

- 1 T smooth peanut butter
- 1/3 cup coconut milk
- 1 t soya sauce
- 1 t fish sauce

For the fridge clean-up BBQ sauce:

- ¼ cup thick soya sauce
- 2 T tomato sauce
- 2 t vinegar
- 2 T peach jam
- 2 t orange juice

For the turmeric noodles:

- Woolworths' prepared garlic, ginger, chili and turmeric
- 2 T vegetable oil

- Woolworths' fresh ready cooked undo noodles
- ½ leftover shredded chicken
- Grated raw baby marrow, for serving
- Sliced spring onions, for serving
- Sesame seeds, for serving

Instructions

4. For the peanut butter dressing, combine 1 T smooth peanut butter, 1/3cup coconut milk, 1 t soya sauce and 1 t fish sauce.
5. For the fridge clean-up BBQ sauce: mix ¼ cup thick soya sauce, 2 T tomato sauce, 2 t vinegar, 2 T peach or apricot jam and 2 t orange juice and simmer for 5 minutes.
6. For the turmeric noodles: place ½ cube each Woolworths' prepared garlic, ginger, chili and turmeric and 2 T vegetable oil in a pan and fry until golden. Toss through warmed leftover noodles or Woolworths' fresh ready cooked undo noodles.
7. To assemble: add ½ leftover shredded chicken to the pan of simmering BBQ sauce and toss to coat. Serve with the warm turmeric noodles, grated raw baby

marrow, sliced spring onions and a sprinkle of sesame seeds or peanuts if you have.

28. Egg Noodle Bowls with Fried Eggs, Bacon, Roast Tomatoes
and Mushrooms

Prep Time: 10 Minutes

Cook Time: 20 Minutes

Servings: 4

Ingredients

- 2 garlic cloves, sliced
- 350 g Woolworths Bella tomatoes, halved
- 1 T olive oil
- 2-3 T Woolworths harissa paste
- 1x 500ml carton Woolworth's organic vegetable stock
- Sea salt and freshly ground black pepper, to taste
- 200 g Woolworths dried egg noodles (or 500g fresh)
- 250 g Woolworths wood-smoked streaky bacon, grilled
- 4 free-range eggs, fried
- Exotic mushrooms, pan-fried, for serving (optional)
- Basil, for serving

Instructions

1. Fry the garlic and tomatoes in the olive oil in a deep pan for 2 minutes. Add 2 T harissa paste and fry for a further minute.
2. Add the stock and 2 cups water. Simmer for 10 minutes and season to taste. Add more harissa if you like.
3. Serve warm with the cooked noodles, bacon and fried eggs, garnished with basil.

29. Cannellini Bean and Bacon Pasta

Prep Time: 15 Minutes

Cook Time: 10 Minutes

Servings: 4

Ingredients

- 500 g spaghetti
- 1 x 400 g cannellini beans, drained
- 125 ml olive oil
- 2 lemons, juiced
- Sea salt and freshly ground black pepper, to taste
- 200 g bacon, roughly chopped
- 20 g parsley, chopped

Instructions

1. Cook the pasta in boiling salted water until al dente.
2. Blend the beans, olive oil and lemon juice until smooth. Season to taste.
3. Fry the bacon in a hot pan until crispy.
4. Toss the sauce through the pasta and serve topped with the bacon and parsley.

30. Fish Finger Butty

Prep Time: 15 Minutes

Cook Time: 15 Minutes

Servings: 6

Ingredients

- 1 x 400 g box Woolworths crumbed fish fingers
- Burger buns, to serve
- Crisp lettuce, to serve
- For the chunky tar tare sauce:
- Gherkins, chopped
- Red onions, chopped
- Hard-boiled eggs, chopped
- Dill, chopped
- Parsley, chopped
- Capers, rinsed and chopped
- Mayonnaise
- Woolworths frozen crinkle cut potato chips, to serve

Instructions

1. Cook frozen fish fingers according to package instructions.

2. Toast burger buns in butter in a pan until golden. Fill the bun with the fish fingers, crisp lettuce and a chunky tart are sauce.

3. For the chunky tar tare sauce, combine chopped gherkins, red onions, hard-boiled eggs, dill, parsley and capers with mayonnaise. Serve with crinkle-cut chips, cooked according to package instructions.